COURTHOUSE
TIME MACHINE

A Short Story
By Trent Parkle

Courthouse Time Machine:
A Short Story by Trent Parkle

To my lovely wife: You are the true love of my life.
Thank you for inspiring me to be the best man I can be.
To my children: You fill my heart with love.

Chapter 1

At age 74, Judge Patrick Jamison was the oldest judge to have ever served on the bench of the Pierce County District Court. By statute, the maximum age for judges was set at 75, so there was a solid chance he would retain the distinction of being the oldest judge ever to serve. At the very least, no one would be older than him since Judge Jamison was pretty sure he could make it to age 75.

It wasn't the money that kept him working. He had long ago qualified for a generous state pension. He was already drawing social security payments. He had waited until age 70, figuring that he was earning enough money as a judge and didn't need early social security benefits. Eventually, there was no reason for him to delay collecting social security payments since his benefits would never increase beyond age 70. He wasn't one to leave money on the table for the government to keep.

He enjoyed the status associated with being a judge. Wearing the black robe, having people stand when he entered the courtroom, and being referred to as "your honor" or "judge" was undeniably a perk of the office. But status wasn't what kept on the bench either.

Mostly, Judge Jamison enjoyed working in the community. He needed a sense of purpose. In his view, being a judge was one of the better ways he could improve his adopted hometown of Tacoma, WA. Although his wife would have preferred to have him available to travel more often, his 30 vacation days per year gave them plenty of time to see the world.

Judge Jamison met his wife in court, nearly 40 years ago. Back then, Judge Jamison was known simply as Patrick. He worked as a prosecutor. Dana, at the time, was a public defender. Patrick was immediately drawn to her passion, brilliance, and stunning good looks. He eventually gathered up the courage to ask her out on a date. She agreed to one date, then another.

Soon the two were inseparable. The couple each notified their respective bosses of the dating relationship. Patrick could hardly have cases against Dana during the day, then share a bed with her at night. Similarly, Dana knew it would, at the very least, appear inappropriate for her to represent clients who were being prosecuted by the man she was sleeping with on her personal time. Patrick would later explain to people, only half-jokingly, that he had to marry her because he sure didn't want to have cases against her. She was just too good a lawyer for him to risk his nearly flawless conviction rate by going up against her as opposing counsel.

Dana had been a successful lawyer for many years. She retired at age 62, like any normal, well-adjusted person. Unlike her husband, she didn't feel compelled to spend her remaining good days participating in the grind of legal work. After retirement, she lived life on her own terms. She had always wanted to be a writer. For the most part, her creative side had been limited by the constraints of the legal system. Unleashed from the chains of conformity, her creative juices produced some classic romance novels, and a few poems. Book critics seemed surprised at her breadth and mastery of various genres, but Patrick had no doubt. Dana was gifted and multitalented. She even managed to have a book crack the NY Times top 10.

Undeniably, Judge Jamison had a good life. But he was not immune to the passage of time. For the most part, his body was holding up well. But the headaches were becoming an unwanted distraction. They had started last year, and only seemed to grow in both severity and frequency. He self-medicated with handfuls of Excedrin, and bottles of red wine, mostly the bold Syrah he favored from Walla Walla, WA. When he could no longer hold the headaches at bay, he reluctantly sought professional help. His doctor prescribed a medication (Qulipta-TM), which was more effective than the over-the-counter drugs he had tried, but often made him nauseous and tired. He tended to avoid taking his medication while at work due to the unpleasant side-effects.

Chapter 2

Judge Jamison handled a variety of cases such as DUI, theft, and simple assaults. District Courts in Washington State only handle misdemeanor and gross misdemeanor offenses. Felonies are handled in Superior Court. Judge Jamison preferred the work in District Court. He held out hope that if the system could intervene in the lives of those who committed low level offenses, they would not graduate to becoming felony offenders.

Judge Jamison's hopes for a better society were more aspirational than the statistics supported. In reality, the best Judge Jamison could do was to be respectful to those in his courtroom, and to follow the law. The volume of cases in District Court assured that he would not be able to take a deep dive into the lives of those who appeared in front of him. At any given time, he had about 500 open cases and most of those cases were "show cause" hearings where he would address violations of probation.

The system was not designed to effectively change behavior. In many ways the system was, intentionally or not, structured to ensure employment for the massive criminal justice system. Police, lawyers, probation officers, jailors, judges, staff, and a growing support system of victim advocates all earned their living off the system. The momentum from this massive system made changing course too hard, so most people accepted the status quo.

Judge Jamison didn't really track numbers. He enjoyed his blissful ignorance and Pollyanna outlook. In spite of this, or maybe because of this ignorance, he was a popular judge. When he first ran for office many years ago, he faced two opponents. Each was well qualified. One was even a former judge. After the primary election reduced the field to the top two, and he found himself with a narrow lead over the former judge.

The remainder of the race for judge was a blur as he prepared for the general election in November. Most candidates for office have a solid group of hard-working committee members. Patrick had a committee of two; himself and his wife Dana. Friends and supporters assisted at some events, but the hard work came from the husband and wife team. Dana designed his media material such as newspaper and magazine advertisements, as well as the door hangers.

Patrick taught himself how to design the campaign's web page (not particularly well), and their oldest son (Patrick Jr) managed the social media. Their younger son Preston, helped set up the campaign tent at the events. Ultimately, the hard work paid off and Patrick won the election by 20 points. Since that election, no one has ever filed against him for judge. He ran unopposed for five separate four-year terms as judge.

22 years after his first election, Judge Jamison found himself still on the bench and still loving the job. The job wasn't hard, except for the emotional trauma of dealing with defendants and victims. Too many defendants were homeless, addicted to drugs, or both. The victims of crime

wanted their own version of justice and grew frustrated at the slow pace of the criminal justice system.

Most days the job was pretty monotonous. The actual mechanics of being a judge were so routine that he could handle the docket in his sleep. It was always the same. Set the record, welcome the participants to court, read rights, take roll, sign continuance orders, and handle an occasional plea. Jury trials were more challenging but after presiding over 200 of them, even that was manageable. Most people would become bored in such an environment, but Judge Jamison had the perfect level of intelligence to handle being a judge. He was neither too dumb to understand the basic concepts of law, nor smart enough to succumb to boredom. His mind focused on each individual case, never drifting off to a happier place. Sitting behind the bench in his courtroom was his happy place.

Chapter 3

It was January 2, 2024. Judge Jamison would remember the day well. Court had been closed the previous day due to the holiday. This was the first day back on the record in which he would have to announce that it was '2024.' In the month leading up to this date, he had signed many continuance orders in which the parties mistakenly requested a new court date in the year '2023.' Judge Jamison would simply change the year to 2024, knowing that this confusion happens every year.

Predictably, the morning docket didn't start exactly at 9:00 am. The defense attorneys needed to speak with their clients. Defendants often don't prioritize discussing the case with their attorney prior to court. The exception is when a defendant is in jail, in which case the defendant will call the defense attorney a dozen times a day wondering why the attorney (who is usually in court) won't call back immediately.

In the event a defendant wants to resolve his case in court, the defense attorney will need a moment to chat with the prosecutor. As Judge Jamison phrased it, "Attorneys need time to take care of attorney business." Always the pragmatist, Judge Jamison didn't interrupt attorneys who needed this time to resolve cases. Every case resolved today meant one more that wouldn't be on his docket next month.

Eventually the attorneys would take care of business, and Judge Jamison's judicial assistant (JA) would come to the judge's chambers and advise him that it was a good time to take the bench. Today was no different. At 9:30 am, his JA knocked on the door of his chambers. Judge Jamison would say in a loud voice "Come on in!" The JA opened the door and told him "They are ready for you."

Judge Jamison smiled and thanked his JA (Alexis). He walked over to the coat rack, pulled his black robe off the hook, put it on and zipped it up. He followed his JA across the hall and she opened the back entrance to the courtroom. This door is used only for the judge and staff. The JA swung open the door and announced, "all rise" and the judge followed her inside. Everyone in the courtroom stood for the judge. Walking toward the bench, the judge smiled and nodded at the crowd before announcing "please be seated." Everyone then took a seat waiting for the judge to start the formal record. The judge sat down in his chair and looked over at the timer to his left. The red LED readout displayed three horizontal lines, before being activated by the judicial assistant. The timer then reflected the correct time of 9:31 am. The microphones fed the sound of voices into the digital recording software loaded onto the JA's computer.

Judge Jamison leaned into his microphone and set the record, "Thank you, I appreciate everyone being here today. This is our pre-trial hearing docket for January 2, 2023." As he announced the wrong year, his brain scrambled, seeming to shift in all directions grasping desperately to find a secure footing inside his head. He could feel pressure building up inside his body and the headache struck in an instant. His vision blurred. He could see the people in the courtroom but their images were vague and ill-defined, appearing more as ghostly apparitions. His skin became moist and clammy. His head sank and he attempted to steady himself on the bench by placing both hands flat on the black bench in front of him. He was nearly overcome with nausea. He was close to passing out. He closed his eyes fearing that he was going to die. A bright light flashed across his eyes. It reminded him of the rotating flashcubes his grandmother used on the top of her Kodak camera. He could still remember how the light burned into his eyes until his eyes could re-adjust. But this was different. This time light seemed to come from the inside of his head rather than outside. Thinking back on stories of people who survived near death experiences, he knew better than to walk toward the light, but what do you do when the light is all around? He could neither walk toward the light nor avoid it. Then, just as quickly as the flash had filled his head, the light was gone.

Chapter 4

Slowly, his head started to clear. The worst of it seemed to be over. The headache washed away in waves, mirroring the beats of his pulse. The nausea subsided. He opened his eyes and took a look around. He recognized the familiar courtroom. He took a deep breath, relieved that he was back to normal. Looking to his left he searched for the LED timer. How long had he been out? It seemed like forever, but given the lack of medical personnel in the courtroom, apparently he hadn't been out for too long.

The red LED timer displayed 9:32 am. Incredibly, his break from reality took almost no time at all. Playing it off like nothing had happened, he looked toward the counsel tables where the attorneys were sitting. He had handled this same docket literally thousands of times and without even thinking about it he asked "Counsel, do we have any matters ready to proceed?" The prosecutor responded, "Your honor, I believe Ms. McKenzie has a matter ready to go." This was a perfectly predictable response, but something was off.

It took the judge a moment to realize that this prosecutor hadn't been assigned to his courtroom for at least six months. And the defense attorney, Ms. McKenzie, hadn't been in his courtroom in nearly a year. Given the turnover at both offices, it was rare for him to have the same prosecutor or public defender for more than a year or two. In the case of Ms. McKenzie, she left the public defender's office last year to explore greener pastures. She was now an associate at a downtown law firm.

Trying to figure out the situation, he quickly connected the dots and understood the reason she was again in his courtroom. "Ms. McKenzie, it is good to see you." She gave him an odd look, then responded "Thanks judge." Judge Jamison followed up with "I appreciate you taking on a pro bono case. Your firm is to be commended for letting you give back to the community." Law firms often encourage their associates to take on cases at little or no cost to indigent clients as part of a commitment to give back to the community.

The young attorney seemed thoroughly confused. Although she was in his courtroom nearly every work day, Judge Jamison had become notoriously forgetful when it came to the names of the attorneys. Maybe he was having a "senior moment" and simply forgot where she worked. Rather than embarrass the judge she responded jokingly, "Well, I guess you *could* call the public defender's office a firm."

Still a bit lost, Judge Jamison risked embarrassing himself and asked her, "Oh, are you back with the public defender's office? Last I heard you had joined a firm downtown." Ms. McKenzie's face turned red, she looked down, and she stammered, "Um, strangely, I recently applied to work at a firm, but I haven't told anyone. Did they reach out to you?"

None of this was making any sense. Judge Jamison looked over at his judicial assistant to see if she also seemed confused. Sitting in the JA chair was Cindy. She had been his JA prior to Alexis. Cindy left the JA position to pursue a supervisor job in the probation department nearly a year ago. Cindy gave the judge a raised eyebrow and waited for some signal that she should stop the record ahead of the judge announcing a recess. No such request came from the judge so she focused on her computer screen.

Judge Jamison wondered to himself if his brain finally broke. Staring ahead at one of the two computer monitors on his bench, something caught his eye. In the lower right hand corner of his computer screen the toolbar displayed the time and date. The time looked right, but something was off about the date. The computer displayed a date of January 2, 2023. Although not a computer expert, Judge Jamison knew that computers didn't simply forget to advance to the new year. So the date was exactly a year behind what it was when he took the bench. He thought to himself, "No fucking way! Have I travelled back in time?" That was the only thing that made sense. But that didn't make sense either. To the best of his knowledge time travel had not yet been invented. But there was no way he had simply imagined an entire year going by.

Apologizing to Ms. McKenzie, he explained that yes, someone had tipped him off about her application to the downtown firm. He told her that he feels good about her chances. He then declared a recess, claiming that he forgot about a quick phone call he needed to make.

The JA again commanded "All rise" and Judge Jamison hastily departed the courtroom and retreated to his chambers. He searched his mind for how any person could verify going back in time. His first stop was to search for the full year calendar he had taped to the back of his chambers door. Every year he taped a new one to the back of his door. Despite having a calendar on this computer, he liked the long physical calendar. When sitting at his desk in his chambers, he just needed to look up and find dates he was looking for at any given time. It was often easier than turning on the computer.

Today, looking at the back side of the door, he found the calendar. The year displayed 2022, which made sense if the date was now January 2, 2023. Judge Jamison knew himself well enough to know that probably wouldn't have taken down the 2022 calendar yet.

He sat down at his desk and took a look at his chambers computer monitors. The screens were locked, but the screen on the left displayed the date of January 2, 2023. Judge Jamison needed to get into his computer to check for some additional verification that he had travelled back in time. He religiously locked his computer when away from his desk. The IT people did random inspections and threatened to impose additional security training classes for anyone who violated the requirement to lock the computer when away. Since he had access to the state criminal database, the State Patrol similarly mandated computer security discipline.

He entered his password to unlock his computer, but his current (2024) password did not work. Trying to remember his code from a year ago, it took him three tries to guess correctly. When the computer opened, he immediately searched through his most recent emails. Like most people, he received about 200 emails per day despite the filters installed by the county IT department. He scrolled to the top of the screen and identified seven new emails received in the morning. All of the emails were dated January 2, 2023. None of the emails were from any date later than January 2, 2023.

He then opened up File Explorer and reviewed documents he had saved to his computer. The most recent documents were dated late December 2022. So, this had really happened. Somehow, he had travelled back in time. Sitting for a moment he tried to digest the seemingly impossible situation in which he found himself. He realized he would probably not be able to determine how it had occurred but he was stuck with the reality that it had occurred. Or maybe he wasn't stuck. Going back in time didn't need to be a bad thing. Maybe this was an amazing opportunity.

Chapter 5

Judge Jamison wondered what he would do now that he had travelled back in time by one year. Having advised the office manager that he was sick and would need coverage for the remainder of his docket that day, he went home to see his wife. On the short drive home, he pondered the opportunities. Gifted with insider knowledge of the year to come, there were ways he could profit financially from time travel. He tried to think of which stocks had gained the most in the last year. Unfortunately he hadn't kept up on the stock market and couldn't think of a sure winner. He knew interest rates had gone up significantly in the last year, but he didn't know how to profit from that either.

Next his mind went to sports. If he knew which teams would win, he could place bets and be guaranteed a win. Superbowl was a month away, and he remembered that the Kansas City Chiefs had narrowly beaten the Philadelphia Eagles in 2023. He couldn't remember the exact score, but remembered it was a fairly high scoring game. He and his wife had cheered frequently, hoping that Patrick Mahomes could pull out the victory, which he did. Betting on the Chiefs, and maybe also betting the over/under would net a profit. Necessarily, that meant he could also place bets for playoff wins for each of the two teams.

Betting was only legal at the Indian Casinos in his state. The Emerald Queen Casino was not far from his home in

Tacoma. His wife was always up for an adventure, and this seemed like a great time to get away with her for the day. He was feeling inexplicably good. He noticed that his headaches seemed to have largely receded. Like a frog in a slowly warming pot, he hadn't fully realized how the severity of his headaches had increased over the last year. He was now feeling better than he had since...well since early 2023.

Arriving at his home in the Northend neighborhood of Tacoma, Judge Jamison slowed his Jeep Wrangler and pointed it up his steep driveway, pausing briefly to push the button on the garage door opener. He and his wife loved their home. Her book sales afforded them an opportunity to live in a beautiful home on a hill, with a pool in the backyard, and a nearly unobstructed 180 degree view of Commencement Bay. Their home was sufficiently large such that opening the garage door did not alert Dana that he was home. He walked through the basement accessed from the attached garage, rounded the corner and walked up the stairs. He assumed he would find Dana in the study, and he assumed correctly.

Sensing movement outside the glass door of the study, Dana looked up startled, placed her hand over her heart, then she recognized her husband approaching. Nearly shouting she said, "You scared the shit out of me!" She frowned for a moment, then the frown softened, and she asked him "Are you OK? Why are you home. I thought you were working today." "Hi lover" he responded with a broad smile. "I was working but I declared myself sick so I could come and see you." She waited a moment for him to explain the real reason why he was home. When no other reason presented itself, her reaction was a combination of confusion and appreciation.

A tear formed in her eye. She knew he loved her and he was never shy about telling her as much, but he was not known for grand romantic gestures. Hardly realizing herself how much she needed a showing of appreciation, she broke down crying. The crying progressed to sobbing. Patrick was shocked, and suddenly he felt ashamed. His failure to meet her needs resulted in Dana bottling up her desires. She had never complained, and always stood by his side. She was always the supportive wife, attending events with him, applauding his successes and consoling him in tough times. She had deserved more from him. And now he had a second chance thanks to the courtroom time machine.

He walked over to her, reached out his hand and helped her up out of her chair. He placed his arms around her and held her tightly. He rubbed his hands on her back slowly and softly, letting her cry until she was done. He whispered "I love you so much!"

Suddenly the trip to the casino seemed so trivial. Sure, she would likely go with him if he asked. But toward what end? Was he really going to waste this day going to a smoke-filled casino just to place bets on football games? He didn't need the money, but he needed his wife to know how much he cares for her, and how important she is to him. The pair released their embrace, and he asked her "How about we pack a couple bags and check into the Four Seasons in Seattle." He knew that was one of her favorite places. They had spent a weekend there nearly three years ago for their anniversary.

In a soft voice, Dana answered "Yes, I would love that. Let's do it!" The two wasted little time and packed overnight bags. Patrick secured a reservation for a room overlooking Elliot Bay. At over $2,000 for the night, the room was not cheap. But he would never regret spending the day with his wife, and making sure she knows that she is important and that he loves her.

They loaded up into his wife's Mercedes GLE. It was a comfortable and luxurious German road vehicle. Less than an hour later, they arrived at the hotel entrance and parked at the valet station. They grabbed their bags and Judge Jamison handed the key to the valet. Walking through the lobby was like entering a different world. The Four Seasons radiates opulence. The marble floors and dark wood trim seemed like something better suited to royalty. He would not be hearing about homelessness or drug addiction today. He was not at work.

Approaching the front desk, the "Guest Relations Consultant" greeted them with a smile. As she processed the guest keys, she asked what brought them to the Four Seasons. Patrick proudly responded that "I am playing hooky so I can spend the day with the love of my life." Looking to his left, his wife's face was beaming. Today she would get some overdue confirmation that she is the most important person in his world.

Chapter 6

The couple managed to secure a room on the eighth floor of the hotel with a spacious suite overlooking Elliot Bay. The weather was atypical for Seattle in the winter. Instead of dark and dreary, the sun made a rare appearance. The room provided a magnificent view of Puget Sound and the Olympic Mountains, the rays of sun danced on the water and showcased the white snow-capped mountains to the northwest.

Patrick ordered room service including a bottle of champagne, Veuve Clicquot that his wife was so fond of drinking on special occasions. And this was truly a special occasion. In court, Judge Jamison often told defendants that it is never too late to do better. Now he was getting a chance to take his own advice. He would do better. He would focus on what really mattered. His wife really mattered.

Waiting for room service, Patrick and Dana re-arranged the chairs, bringing them up to the window, angling them so that their feet could share an ottoman. They both faced the glass window and enjoyed the view. Dana was clearly thrilled that her husband called in sick. He was usually the one who worked through the holidays so that others could have time with their family. While noble, she wished he would sometimes let others cover the holiday dockets so he could spend time with her. Now, without any reason, he ditched work to be with her. This was a welcome change of pace.

Sooner than expected, room service arrived and the waiter knocked on the door. Patrick answered and made room for the food cart which was loaded with champagne and charcuterie. The cart was topped with a white cloth cover, and the charcuterie enjoyed its own stainless steel plate and lid. Always one to be kind to staff, Patrick signed for food and drink and added a generous tip.

Patrick grabbed the bottle and stripped away the foil. He twisted the end of the metal cage and pulled the cork. Slowly, the cork surrendered its grip on the bottle, rewarding the pair with the expected pop. Still holding the cork in his hand, Patrick tilted the bottle and poured two glasses. He handed one to Dana and stretched out his glass toward hers. She did the same and they both said "Cheers!" as the glasses clinked together.

Patrick reached into his overnight bag and grabbed a prescription bottle. In a conspicuous manner gaining Dana's attention, he shook the bottle, twisted the white cap, and pulled out two blue pills. At 74 (73 again now), he could use a little assistance and relied on the magic of the pharmaceutical industry. Dana gave him a grin, laughed, and said "Oh really? What do you have in mind good Sir?" "You will find out in a mere 15-30 minutes." He responded. She laughed again and said jokingly, "I'll start the timer."

A couple glasses of champagne, and about 30 minutes later, the cones and rods in Patrick's eyes sent back unusual signals, causing a bluish/green tint to be added to his otherwise normal vision. This was a sure sign that the blue pills were starting to take effect. He looked over at Dana and smiled. She looked back at him with a sly grin. He grabbed her hand and asked if she would like to join him on the bed.

She said, "No sense in spending all this money and not test out the bed." Agreeing with her compelling argument he walked her over to the end of the bed and pushed her over gently. The clothes came off and the two pulled the covers over their naked bodies. Patrick then demonstrated the other, more traditional effect of the little blue pills.

Later, but not that much later, Patrick asked Dana what she would like to do with their day off. Although it was tempting to put on the soft white bathrobes with the Four Seasons logo and simply lounge in the gorgeous room, Dana wanted to take advantage of their day. Dana responded with a simple answer. "I want to do everything!" Marriage is about compromise, so neither of them tended to get everything they wanted, but Dana had been handed a blank check to plan whatever she wanted. She was going to take advantage of the moment.

The two walked around Seattle. Dana managed to drag Patrick into girly clothing stores, soap and fragrance stores, kitchen stores and a complete tour of Pike Street Market. She even talked him into making dinner reservations at Spinasse, the kind of restaurant that Patrick would generally reject as being overpriced and underwhelming.

Arriving at Spinasse, Dana loved the smell of the authentic Italian dishes and their fragrant spices. The waiter seated them promptly. At the table next to them sat four people, two men and two women. They were a few years younger than Patrick and Dana, and appeared to be friends on something of a double date. Judging from their smiles and laughter, they appeared to be having a good time. They were loud but in a happy way. Their background noise actually made it easier for Patrick and Dana to have a conversation without feeling like the whole restaurant was hanging on their every word.

When the waiter came to take their drink orders, Dana selected a red wine from Italy. Although Patrick really enjoyed drinking wine, Dana had the more refined palette, so he generally deferred to her judgment. They had often talked about taking a trip to Italy but somehow that plan never materialized. Patrick now wished he had made more of an effort to plan the trip with Dana. There were many things he wished he had done better or sooner, but it always seemed like they had unlimited time remaining in their lives.

The restaurant prided itself on their three-course meals, and Patrick and Dana both ordered similar dishes. Patrick liked the food. He had to admit that it was beyond good and well into the realm of delicious. It was still over-priced in his view, but at least he couldn't say it was underwhelming. Dana loved every minute of the experience and every bite of her food.

Patrick asked her about her latest book project. She gave him details about what she had planned. It was going to be a departure from her previous endeavors. She was going to write a non-fiction book covering the history of the Russian ballet. It seemed there was no subject she could not master, and he was proud of her. She had broad interests and enjoyed the pleasure of discovering fine details that others had missed. As she talked, he couldn't help but smile at her. Why had they not done this more often? Looking at his wife, he focused on her beauty. She was a beautiful woman in every visible way, and she also had a beautiful soul.

Eventually, their time at Spinasse came to an end. It came to a natural end because they were done with dinner, but also the restaurant imposed maximum time limits. Business was good, so they needed to clear tables to seat those who had upcoming reservations.

Walking back to the hotel, they held hands. They talked a little on the way, but more than that it was just a time to reflect on their day together. Patrick was pleased that he had not squandered an opportunity to be with the love of his life. She is and was the most important person in the world.

Arriving at the hotel, it had been a full day, and they were both tired. They each took a shower then put on the soft white robes with the hotel logo. They got in bed and turned on some housewives show on Bravo that his wife liked to watch as something of a guilty pleasure. Patrick didn't remember falling asleep, but he was out almost the moment his head hit the pillow.

Chapter 7

Patrick awoke to find himself fully dressed and sitting at his desk in his chambers at work. He had wondered about the limits of time travel. He wasn't sure if he would stay in 2023 or wake up back in his own time. And he didn't know how long he would be away. Now he knew he was only gone a few hours.

Checking the time and date on his computer he confirmed that it was 2024. It was 9:30 am January 2, 2024. His judicial assistant Alexis knocked on the door. Not knowing what kind of universe altering event might transpire if he deviated from the normal script, he answered "Come on in!" and Alexis entered, advising the judge "They are ready for you." The judge responded, "Thank you Alexis, I will be right out."

He needed a moment to figure out his next move. He had so many questions but no one to answer them. Realizing that he travelled back in time, he wondered if he could do it again. And since the first time had been an accident, would the time machine only work if he accidentally said the wrong date, or could he choose a date and go back to that time? He needed a plan, and he needed it quickly.

Assuming he could pick a date, what would he pick? Would he pick a good time or a bad time? He wondered if he could do something good by fixing a historical wrong. Being somewhat self-centered, he wasn't thinking about saving the world. He wasn't going to go back in time, kill Hitler, then stop WWII. In fact, knowing that his last time travel took him to the age he was a year ago, he couldn't select a time before his birth. So then what event during his lifetime could he fix?

Thinking back to the worst moment in his life, he knew what he would like to change. Shortly after his election to judge, Patrick's oldest son Preston joined the Navy. Preston had wanted to serve his country. He had also wanted to follow in his father's footsteps. Patrick had served in the Army for many years, and although he would gently tease Preston for selecting the Navy, he also let him know he was supportive and proud of his decision.

Preston did well in the Navy, advancing quickly. Unknown to Patrick, Preston was battling dark demons in his mind. Although Patrick never learned the exact details, Preston was struggling to deal with something in his past. The structure of the Navy provided him some guard rails, and provided him with a built in support team. But it wasn't enough.

Two years into his enlistment, Preston sat in a folding lawn chair outside the rental home he shared with a couple buddies from the base. He drank his last Dr. Pepper. He placed an M16 under his chin and pulled the trigger. The bullet bounced off the inside of his skull tunnelling through large parts of his brain, never making an exit. Preston died that day while serving in the Navy.

Judge Jamison remembered that day well. It was August 6, 2002. He had been a judge for just two years. During the campaign, Preston had helped him set up the tent, and help with anything else that required the strength of a teenager.

He was strong as an ox, and never shied away from physical exertion.

Preston enjoyed rules and he became frustrated with those who didn't follow rules, and even more frustrated when the system lacked accountability for those who violated the rules. The military seemed like a good fit in that regard. Lots of rules and lots of consequences for breaking rules.

Preston was really smart, but he tended to focus his efforts on subjects which interested him. This inability to focus on boring subjects nearly prevented his graduation from high school. But somehow he barely made it through.

Based on his high ASVAB score, the Navy made a hard push for Preston to sign up for the nuclear program. They offered him nearly $30,000 in enlistment bonuses and dangled the prospect of even more money if he later re-enlisted. But Preston knew what he wanted. He wanted to work with his hands. He wanted to fix jet engines. He rejected the generous enlistment bonus of the nuclear program for the simple reason that he wanted to enjoy his work.

Preston shipped out to Navy Basic Training just two weeks after graduating from high school. He called his dad midway through basic training and let him know that basic training isn't that bad. Thinking he was understating the difficulty of basic training, his dad asked Preston to explain what he meant. Preston explained that when he worked at the grocery store during high school they made him clean the bathrooms nearly all day. The Navy only made him clean toilets part of the day, therefore it wasn't so bad.

Preston went on to become the top graduate in his 'A' school. He was also the top graduate in his 'C' school. His command referred him to a promotion board. The board unanimously recommended him for early promotion. In two years Preston went from E1 to E5, earning the status of non-commissioned officer. To the outside world, Preston appeared to be living his best life.

No parent should have to bury his son. It is not the way of the world for the young to die so early. Patrick hadn't figured out all the angles of time travel, but if there was a way to change the past and prevent Preston's death, Patrick had to try. If it went the same as last time, Patrick would have only 12 or 13 hours to fix the past. That would be enough time to drive to Preston's base at Whidbey Island NAS. It would be enough time to stop him, and help him, or at least find someone who could help him.

Judge Jamison put on his black robe. He knocked twice on the door leading to the back of the courtroom behind the bench. He opened the door and his JA announced "All rise!" Judge Jamison followed the same script, not wanting to change the formula for time travel. He looked around the courtroom, smiled and said, "Please be seated." The time displayed three horizontal dashes before turning on and displaying the correct time of 9:31 am. So far so good.

Judge Jamison announced, "Thank you for being here today. This is our docket for August 6, 2002."

Chapter 8

Like last time, the first effects were a scrambled brain, and blurred vision. Then came the crushing headache, even more severe than the last time he had time travelled. The pain immobilized Judge Jamison. He couldn't brace himself this time, and his head dropped noticeably. He closed his eyes trying to block out the incomprehensible pain and the disturbing streaks of light. Sweat covered his forehead and the rest of his body displayed the sheen from sweat glistening on every exposed surface, as well as everywhere that could not be seen under his robe. He was sure he was going to throw up. The flash inside his head was also brighter and lasted longer.

Then the flash was gone. He opened his eyes. His vision returned to normal. His headache took longer to dissipate but as the seconds ticked by, he was able to regain the use of his mind. But he was still nauseous. He swirled around in his chair and grabbed the black waste basket on the floor. He leaned in and convulsed for a moment before the vomit exploded from his mouth, mostly landing in the waste basket.

Looking up, he saw Gary, his first judicial assistant. Gary looked shocked. Without asking the judge, Gary turned off the recording, telling the courtroom "We are in recess." Judge Jamison muttered "excuse me" and stepped off the bench. He went back to his chambers, this time seeking only a cursory confirmation that he had gone back in time. Gary was on his heels asking if the judge was alright. The obvious answer from Judge Jamison was "No, not at all. Please let, um what's her name, our judicial manager, know that I am sick and need coverage today." Gary responded, "Yes, I will let Susan know you are sick and going home for the day. Take care judge."

Judge Jamison quickly checked his pants pocket to find his car keys. He pulled out a set of Honda keys, and remembered that back in 2002 he was driving a Honda Odyssey minivan. It was a relic from when the kids were younger, but it had come in handy during the election nearly two years prior.

As the headache receded, he noticed that his body was feeling really good. He was 20 pounds lighter than at the start of 2024. Back then, Judge Jamison was competing in triathlons and actually used his YMCA gym membership. It had been a long time since he had a regular work out routine. But this was not a time to enjoy his more fit frame. Patrick needed to focus on the important task at hand.

Judge Jamison considered calling Preston, but he was concerned that changing the past could force Preston to move up his timetable and take his life before his dad could stop him. During his time as judge, Patrick had come to understand that people who really want to commit suicide intentionally avoid reaching out to someone who might try to stop them. It was better to wait until he drove to Preston's rental house off base. He wanted to see Preston in person and stop him from killing himself.

Patrick left the courthouse parking lot and headed toward Whidbey Island. He considered calling Dana to let her know the situation, but he wasn't sure that was a good idea. There was just no way to explain that he found a time machine in his courtroom and had travelled back in time over 20 years to save their son Preston. She might think he was crazy. She might try to stop him, thinking that he had lost his mind and needed medical assistance.

For his part, Patrick was also having trouble digesting the fact that he had travelled through time. And now he had done it a second time. Part of his mind resisted the idea that this had happened at all. There must be another explanation. Maybe he had lost his mind. A look out the window at the heavy I-5 traffic assured him that this was not a fantasy.

The drive to Whidbey Island Naval Air Station was going to take about three hours, assuming the Ferry in Mukilteo was not backed up or out of order. About this time, he wished that the time machine had some kind of directional control. Why did he always need to go back in time to the exact same location?

Setting aside the question of directional time travel for a moment, he focused on his driving. Cursing the seemingly omnipresent Seattle area traffic, Patrick made slower progress than he would have preferred. 90 minutes later he finally made it to the ferry in Mukilteo. Thankfully it was running on schedule, and he was able to drive on to the lower-level vehicle parking section about ¾ of the way back on the ferry. Once onboard, he exited his vehicle, but only because safety regulations require that he not stay in his car. He considered getting a coffee from the small cafeteria on the boat but grabbed a water instead. Despite the gravity of the situation, he was not prepared to drink cafeteria coffee.

Thirty minutes later he arrived at Whidbey Island and departed the ferry along with a row of twenty cars ahead of him. At this time of day, Preston would not be at his rental house, and Judge Jamison didn't want to wait. He decided to make his way directly to the base and find Preston.

He took the short drive to the Naval Air Station and was stopped by the gate guard. Judge Jamison was still a reservist in the Army and had a valid military ID identifying him as a Captain. He hoped the gate guard was not going to ask him to explain the purpose of his visit. The only option in that case would be to lie. The gate guard saluted when he examined Judge Jamison's ID, and said "Welcome to Whidbey Island NAS, Sir." The judge returned the salute and thanked the guard. He considered asking the guard for directions but decided that he was lucky enough to be on base and he didn't want to give the gate guard time to second guess granting him access.

Judge Jamison didn't know the exact unit where he would find Preston but eventually he found his way to the welcome center. Judge Jamison explained to the sailor manning the front desk that he needed to find his son, and that his son was experiencing emotional distress and needed assistance immediately. He didn't know Preston's exact unit, but explained that he works on jet engines for the P8 Poseidon and was part of the "Skinny Dragons."

Judge Jamison expected a great deal of resistance but was met instead with a great deal of assistance. He was met by the Navy's version of a Military Police, called MA's. Having been advised of the situation by the front desk, the MA called ahead to Preston's unit and asked to have Preston available for Judge Jamison. The MA allowed the judge to follow him to Preston's unit where, upon arrival, a grumpy looking Gunnery Sergeant "greeted" him by asking "what the hell is this all about?"

Judge Jamison explained that Preston was in a state of emotional distress. "I am concerned for his safety. Preston is planning a life ending event." Back in 2002, the military was hesitant to recognize suicide as being a legitimate problem. Judge Jamison hoped to soften the blow by calling it a life-ending event. Unfortunately, this choice of words could also mean that Preston was planning to kill someone else. This got their attention, so the judge didn't offer any clarification.

By this time, Preston had been called out of the machine shop where he was working. They brought him to his father. Judge Jamison gave Preston a big hug and got to say all the things he had wanted to say before his son took his own life. He told him that help is available and he doesn't have to face his demons alone. Preston was initially shaking his head and looking at his father like he was crazy. Then his eyes watered up. He asked his dad how he knew. Absent an answer that made sense, his father told him "Dads just know these things." He gave Preston a big hug and told him it would be alright and that he loves him.

The grumpy gunny changed his demeanor. Judge Jamison asked him what kind of mental health services they have on base. The gunny sheepishly replied that they have a medical doctor to examine most mild physical ailments but they were kind of limited on the mental health side. "But, we do contract with the county for a Designated Crisis Responder (DCR)." He offered to call the Island County DCR, and Judge Jamison said "yes, please." Preston said flatly "No way!"

Preston was in a tough spot. If the DCR determined that Preston was in danger of harming himself or others, the Navy would strip him of access to weapons. The ability to carry weapons is a requirement of military service. This defining moment could end Preston's military career. Having the benefit of seeing the future, the judge knew Preston would be facing a far worse consequence than losing his job unless someone intervened. This was a no brainer.

"Look Gunny, you have just heard Preston admit that he is not well. He needs help. He is too proud or strong to ask for help but he needs it. If you can't make this happen, I will need a word with the base commander." Judge Jamison wasn't going to take no for an answer. Gunny figured he better call the commander anyway. This was quickly escalating above his pay grade.

Gunny picked up the land line and placed a call. The judge could hear Gunny's end of the conversation. He explained that Preston's dad, CPT Jamison, insists that we have DCR evaluate Petty Officer Jamison out of concern that he is at risk for committing a life ending act."

Gunny had used Judge Jamison's military rank, not specifying that the judge is an Army CPT, and a reservist at that. There are also Captains in the Navy, but their rank structure is different. A Navy Captain is an O-6, which is the equivalent of a Colonel in the Army. An Army Captain is only an O-3. The base commander was left with the impression that he and Judge Jamison held the same military rank. Judge Jamison could picture what the base commander told the gunny based on the shortness of the conversation. Gunny said, "Yes Sir. I will do that, we will get the DCR over here ASAP, or we will escort Petty Officer Jamison to the county for an evaluation."

Preston was not happy with his father, but also seemed relieved. He didn't have to fight alone. As Gunny made arrangements, Judge Jamison asked if he could escort his son to the evaluation. Holding up one finger as if to signal for the judge to wait a moment, Gunny continued to talk on the phone, taking notes and discussing the situation with the DCR. After a short and efficient phone conversation, Gunny let the judge know that he would not be able to escort his son on the trip to the DCR. The DCR insisted that Preston be evaluated overnight on a mental health hold. The judge gave his son a big hug and again said "I love you Preston." He promised to come up and visit Preston over the weekend. He watched as Preston loaded up into the police car, which seemed far better than a ride in a funeral hearse.

Judge Jamison pulled open the door and got back in the minivan. He sat in the plush leather seats and could finally relax for a moment. He closed his eyes and thought about how lucky he was to have a chance to fix a terrible wrong. Preston deserved a second chance. He deserved to live.

Chapter 9

Judge Jamison opened his eyes and he was back in his chambers. He checked the time and date. It was 9:30 am, January 2, 2024. Thinking back on his second travel back in time, it was much shorter than the first. His JA knocked on the door, and the judge said "Come on in!" His JA told him "They are ready for you." "I will be right out" replied the judge.

The headache was back like it had a vendetta against him, and he wasn't even on the bench yet. He needed a plan. He had no idea how long the time machine would be up and running, but he didn't want to waste the opportunity. After he saved Preston, he needed something a little lighter. Thinking back, he wanted to return to his favorite time in recent memory.

For their anniversary nine years ago, he and Dana took a vacation to Maui. They flew first class. They stayed at an expensive condo on the water. They had a great time and enjoyed each other's company. He wanted to go back there, and he wanted to be with Dana.

Getting up out of his chair in his chambers, he grabbed the black robe, put it on, and zipped it up. He knocked twice on the door leading to the back of the courtroom. He cringed and tried to power through the headache, and said "Please be seated." He looked across the courtroom. He wondered if it was worth the effort to try to time travel again. Last time nearly destroyed his brain. But he wanted to give it one more try. He announced "Thank you, I appreciate everyone being here today. This is our docket for September 3, 2014."

He no sooner uttered the date than his body went into convulsions. His brain felt like someone detonated a grenade somewhere between his ears. His vision went dark except for the trail of light coming from nowhere. He closed his eyes, needing to focus on ordering the pain to leave him. He could feel his head slip down on the bench. He pissed himself and needed to throw up. The light would have blinded him if it came from outside his head. Finally, when he feared he would not make it another moment, he started to come out of the death spiral.

Chapter 10

Unlike the first two times, this time it took longer for him to regain anything remotely close to consciousness. And unlike the other times, he did not wake up at his bench in the courtroom. He could feel something warm on his skin. The bright light now seemed to be coming from outside his eyes. He could hear a dull noise in the background. The smell was different. It was sea air. As he slowly opened his eyes, he realized the bright light was the sun making its way through his Ray-Bans. The sounds in the background were the waves crashing just a few feet from his lounge chair. He looked to his right and saw the love of his life. Dana was right next to him. She was also in a lounge chair. She was reading a paperback book, shaded by her wide brimmed straw hat.

He was back in Maui! And he was with his wife. The warm air relaxed his body, and his headache started to clear, but he was so tired. Summoning what little strength he had, he stretched his right arm over and touched her hand. He told her "You are the most important person in the world to me!" She said "Ahhhh, I love you so much!"

He was so tired, but he managed to sit up in his chair. He reached down to grab the aluminum cup he brought down from the condo. The cup had a plastic top with a slider which was closed now to prevent sand from blowing into his drink. The cup reminded him of an adult sippy cup. He remembered his own young kids drinking out of cups which were nearly identical to his cup. But his cup was filled with a Mai Tai. He and Dana had mixed up the light and dark rum along with pineapple juice and ice. They had enjoyed many of these drinks while in Maui.

He pushed open the slider on the cup and took a long pull of the tropical drink. It was cool and refreshing. He rum had a bit of a kick. He obviously had been heavy handed when mixing the drink. Even so, a smile crossed his face.

Back in 2014 he had considered cancelling the trip to Maui. He was so busy at work. The never-ending stack of files kept growing on his desk. Plus, he had trials coming up that he needed to prepare. It was Dana who convinced him that the work will always be there. She told him "You need a vacation. And frankly so do I."

Sitting on the beach in one of the most beautiful places on earth, he couldn't imagine what he had been thinking. He was relieved that the 2014 version of himself had not cancelled the trip. At this moment there was no place he would rather be and no one he would rather be with than his wife. Dana took off her hat and set down her book. She stood up and told Patrick, "I am going to take a dip. Care to join me?" He was tired, but he really wanted to follow her into the water. He smiled and told her, "You bet! Let's go."

The water was a turquoise blue that the Hawaiian Islands were famous for, and the water temperature was about 80 degrees. Along with a chance to be with his wife, getting in the water seemed irresistible. He joined her in the warm sea, and they waded out until the gentle waves hit them at chest level. Patrick remembered what he liked so much about this memory. It was a rare time when all of the stress of his life evaporated away.

He didn't have any need to save the world out here. He didn't need to think about his duties as a judge. He didn't need to determine who went to jail or who got a second chance. All he needed was his wife, warm blue water, and a drink waiting for him back at his lounge chair.

Dana smiled, seeming to read his mind. She knew she was right to insist that they get away to Maui. They needed to bank memories and experiences. Life is too short to work all the time. She waded toward him and gave him a hug and a kiss. He lifted her out of the water and spun her around teasingly. She laughed and wrapped her legs around his hips. A large wave knocked them off balance and washed over the couple. They were having fun, content to enjoy each other's company.

Walking back to the lounge chairs, Patrick grabbed a towel and dried his chest and swimsuit. Placing the towel back on the chair, he sat down and leaned back. Unable to keep his eyes open, he again drifted off to sleep.

Chapter 11

His next memory was that of another bright light crossing his closed eyes. This light came from the outside rather than inside his head. But he couldn't seem to open his eyes. His ears began to activate gradually like they were on a dimmer switch. He began to hear muffled voices. Listening closely, he heard the buzzing and beeping of machinery. He struggled to make out the voices in the background.

He could hear the voice of a man explaining something complicated. He tried to tune in and focus on the voice. At first it was garbled gibberish, but then it was coming in clearer. He could pick out the man saying "Mrs. Jamison, as you can see from the MRI, the neoplasm in the brain continues to expand rapidly. The tumor has become aggressive and inoperable. Given the advanced stage of the cancer, it is too late for chemotherapy and radiation. We are trying to keep him comfortable. The pain is likely excruciating but your husband has not gained consciousness in over a week, so we are not sure how much he can feel. Frankly, I am not sure how he managed work as a judge for so long. Commonly, people with a cerebral tumor of this size experience significant degradation of their mental faculties."

Patrick could hear Dana respond to the man telling him, "Thank you doctor. Do you have an idea how much longer he has to live?" The doctor responded, "Sadly, not long. Frankly, you should consider saying your last goodbyes."

Pushing back the tears in her eyes, she looked at her husband's face. He had done a good job of covering up his condition. Maybe if he had done a better job of seeking help, he could have lived longer. But having been married to him for so long, she knew he tended to understate problems, and focus on what made them happy. It would be inconceivable for him to let himself waste away slowly. He wouldn't put her through that, nor would he wish that upon himself. He had undoubtedly known that he was dying long before he lost consciousness in his courtroom sitting on the bench last week.

She squeezed his hand. It was his 75th birthday. She knew that he was always a competitive person, and he would be pleased to know that no sitting judge would ever be older than him. One last victory in a life filled with far more good times than bad.

She thanked the doctor again, then went back to talking to her husband. She had been in the middle of a story about their trip to Maui back in 2014 before the doctor interrupted. Patrick seemed to like that story. Although he was unconscious, she could swear that his lips curled into something resembling a smile.

Judge Jamison tried hard to concentrate but his mind wandered. He wanted to see his wife. He wanted to thank her for being so good to him, and for being such a wonderful person. Despite his efforts, he could not open his eyes.

Dana reached over and held his hand while she continued to tell him about their favorite times together. Her voice was soft and comforting. For a moment, he was at peace. Then the crushing headache returned. It had found him. It brought with it the disorienting light. His mind struggled to find a solace that was not available for him.

The red LED display in the hospital room reflected Patrick's pulse. As the number dropped, a loud alarm blared. A nurse scurried into the room. She checked the many displays which monitored the vital signs of the expiring judge. She called for a doctor. The numbers continued to drop. By the time the doctor arrived, the number on the red LED display hit zero. A few moments later, three red horizontal dashes replaced the numbers on the display. The doctor announced, "Time of death, 9:31 am, January 10, 2024." Judge Jamison's time on this earth had come to an end.

---THE END---